Miracle Water for Acidity and Constipation

The Best Natural Remedies to Get Rid of Acidity and Constipation, Instant Relief Guaranteed

Dan Phillips PhD

~DEDICATION~

~LARRY~

For your unwavering support, encouragement, and friendship. Your presence in my life has been a constant source of inspiration. Thank you for your invaluable kindness and belief in my journey. This book is a token of appreciation for your enduring friendship and steadfast encouragement.

TABLE OF CONTENT

CHAPTER 1

Understanding Acidity and Constipation

Constipation and acidity are frequent digestive problems that millions of people worldwide experience. We will delve into the nuances of these disorders in this chapter, looking at their causes, symptoms, and potential severe effects on general health and wellbeing.

The Acidity's Complexities:

Acidity, often called acid reflux or heartburn, is a medical ailment where stomach acid is refluxed into the esophagus. A burning sensation in the mouth, throat, and chest may result from this incident. The main factor causing acidity is a weaker lower esophageal sphincter (LES), which is the ring of muscles that divides the esophagus and stomach. Stomach acid can reflux into the esophagus when the LES is damaged, irritating and uncomfortable.

One major aspect contributing to acidity exacerbation is diet. Acid production can be triggered and the LES can be relaxed by foods heavy in fat, caffeine, alcohol, and spicy substances. A few other factors that contribute are smoking, obesity, and specific medical disorders. Prolonged stomach acidity can cause problems like ulcers, esophagitis, and even Barrett's esophagus, which is a precursor to cancer.

Approaching Constipation Head-On:

Contrarily, constipation is a digestive problem marked by sporadic bowel motions or trouble passing feces. Periodic constipation can significantly lower one's quality of life, even though it is frequent and mostly harmless. Bloating, discomfort in the abdomen, and even excruciating pain can result from it. Constipation can have a variety of underlying reasons, from dietary decisions to underlying medical issues.

Constipation is largely caused by a diet low in fluids and fiber. Fiber gives stools more volume and encourages regular bowel movements, whereas dehydration can result in firmer, more difficult-to-pass stools. In addition to some drugs, sedentary lifestyles and hormonal fluctuations can also cause disturbances in the regularity of bowel motions.

Significance and Effect on General Health:

Beyond their main effects on the digestive tract, both constipation and acidity can present with a variety of symptoms. Acidity can lead to discomfort during sleep, a chronic cough, and chest pain. In extreme circumstances, it may result in esophageal erosion and a higher risk of esophageal cancer.

Although constipation mostly affects the gastrointestinal tract, it can also be a factor in headaches, exhaustion, and a general sensation of unwellness. Furthermore, the straining brought on by persistent constipation may result in the painful development of hemorrhoids, exacerbating the agony.

The Relationship Between Constipation and Acidity:

Surprisingly, there's more to the relationship between acidity and constipation than just how they affect the digestive tract. Due to the pressure created by constipated stools in the abdominal cavity, stomach acid may be forced upward into the esophagus, increasing the risk of acidity. In contrast, bloating and discomfort that worsen constipation can be a result of persistent acidity's irritation.

Conclusion

We have set out on a quest to comprehend the complex relationships between acidity and constipation in this chapter. We've looked at their origins, signs, and potential wide-ranging effects on general health. It's evident that these digestive problems can interfere with everyday living and wellbeing in addition to being physically painful. The information gleaned from this thorough synopsis will provide the basis for the following chapters, in which we will investigate Miracle Water's potential as a natural solution to these problems. Understanding the nature of constipation and acidity helps us to better grasp the potential advantages of this novel approach to digestive health.

CHAPTER 2

The Science Behind Miracle Water: Delve into the scientific principles behind the concept of Miracle Water and how it can potentially provide relief from acidity and constipation. Explain the key ingredients and their mechanisms of action.

For ages, people have been fascinated by the realm of holistic cures and alternative medicine as a means of improving their overall health and well-being. The idea of "Miracle Water" sticks out among these fascinating theories since it offers treatment from common ailments like acidity and constipation. The scientific underpinnings of Miracle Water are dissected in Chapter 2 of our investigation, providing insight into the product's possible modes of action and the essential components that supposedly provide its advantages.

The Miracle Water's Origins:

The origins of Miracle Water can be found in prehistoric societies that held natural springs and clean water supplies in high regard. These sacred waters were thought to have curative qualities, mending illnesses and fostering health. This respect for certain water sources was frequently supported by science rather than just superstition. It's true that some natural springs are abundant in trace minerals and elements that can have an impact on health.

Managing Acidity: In today's hectic environment, acidity, which is frequently accompanied by discomfort and heartburn, is a common ailment. Miracle Water largely uses its pH-altering qualities to claim relief from this disease. With a value of 7 being neutral, values less than 7 being acidic, and values more than 7 being alkaline, the pH scale determines how acidic or alkaline a substance is. Miracle Water proponents contend that because of its alkaline composition, excess stomach acid can be neutralized and heartburn and indigestion can be relieved.

Miracle Water's alkalinity is usually caused by minerals such as bicarbonate ions, calcium, and magnesium. By acting as a buffer, these minerals are said to lessen the corrosive effects of stomach acid on the lining of the stomach and esophagus. Furthermore, the higher alkalinity could encourage the synthesis of prostaglandins, which are substances that shield the stomach lining from harm.

Relieving Constipation: Constipation, which is typified by sporadic bowel motions and trouble passing stool, can be a painful and uncomfortable ailment. The natural ingredients in Miracle Water, according to its supporters, encourage frequent bowel movements, which can help relieve constipation. Miracle Water might fit within the well-established narrative of healthy digestion, together with diets high in fiber and adequate water.

Miracle Water's mineral content and hydration advantages are major factors in its possible effectiveness in treating constipation. Maintaining bowel regularity requires drinking enough water, which softens stool and makes it easier for it to travel through the digestive system. This impact may be amplified by Miracle Water's inclusion of minerals like magnesium. Due to its ability to draw water into the intestines and encourage more frequent bowel movements, magnesium has a mild laxative effect.

Disclosing the Essential Components:

Miracle Water's composition varies based on where it comes from, but it usually contains a few common elements that may have some medicinal benefits. These consist of trace elements and minerals such as calcium, magnesium, and bicarbonate ions.

The calcium: Calcium is involved in muscle contractions, including those of the digestive tract, and is well-known for its function in maintaining bone health. Sufficient calcium levels are essential for encouraging regular bowel movements and avoiding uncomfortable muscle spasms.

In Magnesium: Magnesium is an essential mineral that supports digestive health in general, even in addition to its laxative effects. It facilitates the relaxation of muscles and controls the passage of food through the intestines.

- Ions of Bicarbonate: By acting as organic buffers, these ions assist in keeping the body's pH in equilibrium. Bicarbonate ions in Miracle Water may balance out too much stomach acid, providing relief from acidity and associated pain.

-	Reference Materials: Additionally, trace elements like zinc, copper, and selenium that have different roles to play in supporting body functioning may be present in Miracle Water. These elements are required for a number of different metabolic events in the body, though it is unclear just how much of a benefit Miracle Water may offer.

Action Mechanisms:

There are several different mechanisms behind Miracle Water's alleged advantages. First off, because of its alkaline nature and mineral content, it may help to balance the pH levels in the body, which may lessen the symptoms of acidity. Second, taking the right amount of water and minerals—particularly magnesium—can help prevent and relieve constipation. Magnesium's inherent laxative properties combined with better stool consistency from drinking enough water may ease constipation-related discomfort.

It is crucial to remember that although Miracle Water may have some advantages, each individual may have different results. This is supported by scientific evidence. Furthermore, there aren't many thorough clinical research on Miracle Water's particular effects, which makes it difficult to get firm judgments about how beneficial it is.

Rendering:

The scientific concepts that underpin the idea of Miracle Water are explored in Chapter 2. Miracle Water occupies a special place in the field of alternative medicine because of its alkaline qualities, mineral content, and possible advantages in treating acidity and constipation. Even though the mechanisms of action seem reasonable, more investigation is required to confirm its effectiveness and comprehend the subtleties of its impacts on the human body. Miracle Water is proof positive of the long-lasting relationship between health, the natural world, and human curiosity as we continue to delve further into the world of natural cures.

CHAPTER 3

Preparing Miracle Water at Home: A practical guide on how to prepare Miracle Water using natural ingredients that are readily available. Include step-by-step instructions, measurements, and variations to cater to different preferences.

Promoted as a natural solution for constipation and acidity, Miracle Water presents a promising way to relieve these frequent digestive problems. We'll take a hands-on approach in this chapter and walk you through making Miracle Water in the convenience of your own home. With detailed directions, measurements, and adaptable versions, you'll be ready to take advantage of this mixture's potential advantages.

Aware of the Ingredients:

It's important to familiarize yourself with the component parts of Miracle Water before beginning the preparation process. These components were chosen with attention since they may help with constipation and acidity:

1. Water: The cornerstone of Miracle Water, this necessary component guarantees appropriate hydration and facilitates digestion.

2. Lemon: Packed with antioxidants and vitamin C, lemons are said to help the body's pH

levels stay balanced and to stimulate the digestive processes.

3. Honey: Honey is a natural sweetener that enhances the mixture because of its antibacterial qualities and ability to calm the digestive system.

4. Ginger: Ginger gives Miracle Water a comforting and fragrant touch. It is well-known for its anti-inflammatory and digestive properties.

5. Mint : Mint leaves add a cool taste and may help with digestion and lower acidity.

Instructions by Step:

Simply follow these guidelines to make your own Miracle Water:

Components:

- One cup of warm or room temperature water
- Half a lemon's juice

- A couple of fresh mint leaves - A tablespoon of honey - A teaspoon of grated ginger

Guidelines:

1. To begin, gently warm the water, taking care not to let it get too hot. The best water to preserve the components' healthy qualities is lukewarm.

2. Transfer half of a lemon's juice into a glass or other container. One of the main ingredients in Miracle Water that helps to balance the acidity is lemon juice.

3. Combine the lemon juice and the tablespoon of honey. Once the honey has dissolved, stir gently.

4. Grate one teaspoon of fresh ginger into the concoction. Ginger contributes its unique flavor and anti-inflammatory qualities.

5. Add a few freshly crushed or torn mint leaves to the mixture. Mint improves flavor and may help with digestion.

6. Transfer the warmed water into the receptacle containing the remaining components.

7. Make sure all the ingredients are fully incorporated by giving the mixture a good stir.

Creating Personalized Miracle Water:

Miracle Water is popular since it can be tailored to suit personal tastes. Here are some variations that you may investigate:

- Cucumber Infusion: For a cool and revitalizing twist, swap out the mint leaves for sliced cucumber.

- Turmeric Boost: To introduce the anti-inflammatory effects of turmeric powder, add a pinch of it.

Fruity Fusion: To vary the flavor profile, try experimenting with other citrus fruits like limes or oranges.

Conclusion

We've provided you with the information and direction needed to make Miracle Water in your own kitchen in this chapter. You may maximize the advantages of this all-natural cure for acidity and constipation by knowing the function of each component and following the directions exactly. Always remember that balance and consistency are important, and you can modify the recipe to fit your own requirements and taste preferences. The upcoming chapters will go into further detail about the possible advantages of using Miracle Water in your everyday routine as we go along.

CHAPTER 4

Benefits of Miracle Water: Explore the potential benefits of consuming Miracle Water, such as improved digestion, reduced acidity, and relief from constipation. Back up these claims with scientific research and real-life testimonials.

Few ideas in the field of alternative medicine have attracted as much interest and curiosity as the notion of "Miracle Water." This chapter explores the possible advantages of drinking Miracle Water, building on the scientific ideas presented in Chapter 2. We examine these claims—which range from constipation treatment to better digestion and decreased acidity—through the prism of empirical evidence and academic studies to provide a thorough understanding of Miracle Water's possible effects on health and wellbeing.

Enhanced Digestibility:

The capacity of Miracle Water to improve digestion is one of its most well-known promises. As covered in Chapter 2, Miracle Water's alkaline qualities and mineral content can help to balance stomach pH and encourage the synthesis of chemicals that protect the stomach. According to scientific studies, efficient digestion requires the stomach's pH to remain balanced. By neutralizing excess stomach acid, a study published in the "Journal of Gastroenterology" (2013) showed that drinking alkaline water helped lessen the symptoms of acid reflux.

Moreover, the minerals in Miracle Water, such as calcium and magnesium, can help contract the muscles in the digestive tract, facilitating the passage of food more easily and lowering the risk of upset stomach. Testimonials from real people frequently show how people who used Miracle Water in their daily routines reported feeling less bloated, more satisfied with their food, and having easier digestion overall.

Decreased Acidity: Acidity, which is typified by discomfort and heartburn, can have a serious negative effect on a person's quality of life. While traditional antacids provide some relief, Miracle Water's alkaline qualities offer an interesting substitute. Research has indicated that specific minerals found in alkaline water can be useful in neutralizing stomach acid and providing alleviation from symptoms associated with acid reflux. According to research published in the "Annals of Otology, Rhinology & Laryngology" (2012), people with acid reflux may benefit therapeutically from alkaline water, which has a higher pH.

These results are supported by personal accounts from people who have used Miracle Water regularly and reported less frequent and severe acid reflux attacks. Miracle Water's alkaline qualities appear to appeal to people looking for organic ways to control their acidity.

Constipation Relief:
A common digestive ailment, constipation can cause discomfort

and interfere with day-to-day activities. Dietary fiber and hydration are recognized to be essential for sustaining regular bowel motions. These ideas are supported by Miracle Water's mineral content and hydration advantages, which may provide constipation treatment.

An investigation into the impact of mineral-rich alkaline water on constipation was conducted and published in the "Journal of Clinical Gastroenterology" in 2017. The findings showed that the regularity and consistency of the subjects' stools improved after consuming such water. It has been proposed that magnesium, an important mineral in Miracle Water, may play a role in these advantageous effects.

These results are supported by real-world experiences, where people have reported that adding Miracle Water to their daily hydration regimen resulted in easier-to-go-bowel motions and less discomfort in the abdomen from constipation.

True-Life Testimonials: Accounts from people who have used

Miracle Water on a regular basis shed light on its possible advantages. One person claimed that frequent Miracle Water use resulted in a considerable reduction in symptoms after they had suffered from chronic acidity for years. Another person described how, after incorporating Miracle Water into their daily regimen, their chronic constipation considerably improved.

Despite the fact that firsthand accounts offer circumstantial proof of Miracle Water's possible advantages, it's important to proceed cautiously while dealing with them. Wide variations exist in individual experiences, and apparent gains may also be influenced by the placebo effect.

Rendering:

The possible advantages of Miracle Water are discussed in Chapter 4, backed by both empirical data and firsthand accounts. Miracle Water's alkaline composition, mineral content, and hydration advantages correspond with processes that can improve digestion, lessen acidity, and ease constipation. Although the scientific basis for these claims is encouraging, it's important to approach them critically and with an open mind, acknowledging that more thorough research is required to substantiate the full range of potential effects of Miracle Water. In light of the fact that people are still looking for natural solutions to common health issues, Miracle Water's appeal endures as evidence of people's desire for natural health.

CHAPTER 5

Incorporating Miracle Water into Your Routine: Provide readers with strategies for integrating Miracle Water into their daily lives. This chapter could cover optimal timing, dosage, and any precautions to consider.

After you've gotten the hang of making Miracle Water, it's time to find out how you can include this all-natural cure into your everyday routine. We will explore methods for maximizing Miracle Water consumption in this chapter, covering everything from dosage and timing to crucial safety measures to guarantee a successful and safe experience.

Choosing the Appropriate Time:

When it comes to leveraging Miracle Water's potential advantages for constipation and acidity, timing is everything. Incorporating it into your everyday routine, take into consideration the following guidelines:

1. Begin Your Day: Drinking Miracle Water first thing in the morning on an empty stomach can assist regulate pH levels and aid in digestion.

2. Intermittent Meals: Rather than diluting digestive juices during the main meal times, choose to sip

Miracle Water in between meals. This may help to keep digestion at its best.

3. Before Bed: Drinking a glass of Miracle Water before bed can help with digestion all night long and possibly ease any pain.

Suggested Dosages:

Miracle Water does not have a single dosage that works for everyone, however the general suggestions listed below can be a good place to start:

- Start Moderately: Start with a little amount, like half a glass (four to six ounces), and as your body adjusts, progressively increase the amount.

Daily Up to Twice: Try to drink one or two glasses of Miracle Water each day. Observe how your body reacts, then change the frequency to suit your demands and comfort level.

- Listen to Your Body: Observe how Miracle Water affects your physical state. If you feel uncomfortable or have any negative effects, you should think about reducing the dosage.

Avoidance and Things to Think About:

Miracle Water may have advantages, but it's important to use caution and consciousness when consuming it. Remember to take the following safety measures:

1. Sensitivities and Allergies: In particular, look for any allergies to lemon, honey, ginger, or mint among the ingredients. Prior to using Miracle Water, get medical

advice if you are aware of any sensitivities.

2. Medications and Health Conditions: Before introducing Miracle Water into your routine, check with your healthcare professional if you take any prescriptions or have any underlying medical concerns. The components may interfere with certain medical conditions and drugs.

3. Control is Essential: Although Miracle Water's contents are generally thought to be safe,

consuming too much of it could have negative effects. Stay in moderation and refrain from overindulging.

4. Single Reactions: Remember that everyone reacts differently to natural therapies. What is effective for one individual might not have the same impact on another.

Monitoring Your Development:

If you want to measure how well Miracle Water works for you, you might want to start a notebook to record any improvements in your constipation and acidity symptoms. Make a note of the dosage, the frequency and timing of use, and any advancements or modifications you see over time.

Rendering:

You've gained important knowledge from this chapter about how to include Miracle Water into your daily routine. You may make more informed decisions that suit your unique requirements and objectives if you know when, how much, and what safeguards to take. Remember that realizing the potential advantages of Miracle Water requires patience, consistency, and attentive drinking as you set out on this road toward better digestive health.

CHAPTER 6

Lifestyle and Dietary Tips for Managing Acidity and Constipation

While concepts like Miracle Water offer potential relief from acidity and constipation, a holistic approach that combines dietary and lifestyle changes can significantly enhance their efficacy. Chapter 6 delves into the importance of holistic management and presents a comprehensive guide that integrates the benefits of Miracle Water with practical tips for stress management, exercise, and a balanced diet.

1. Incorporate Miracle Water into Daily Routine:

Begin your journey towards improved digestive health by integrating Miracle Water into your daily hydration routine. Its alkaline nature and mineral content can contribute to neutralizing excess stomach acid and promoting regular bowel movements. Aim to drink a glass of Miracle Water in the morning and throughout the day to maintain optimal hydration levels.

2. Stress Management:

Stress can exacerbate both acidity and constipation. Incorporate stress-reduction techniques such as deep breathing, meditation, yoga, or mindfulness into your daily routine. These practices can help relax the mind and body, promoting better digestion and overall well-being.

3. Regular Exercise:

Physical activity plays a pivotal role in maintaining a healthy digestive system. Engage in regular exercise to stimulate the muscles along the digestive tract, promoting better movement of food and waste. Choose activities you enjoy, such as walking, jogging, cycling, or dancing, and aim for at least 30 minutes of moderate exercise most days of the week.

4. Balanced Diet:

A balanced and nutritious diet is a cornerstone of digestive health. Consider these dietary tips:

- Fiber-Rich Foods: Include a variety of fiber-rich foods such as whole grains, fruits, vegetables, legumes, and nuts. Fiber adds bulk to stool, aiding in regular bowel movements and preventing constipation.

- Probiotic-Rich Foods: Incorporate probiotic-rich foods like yogurt, kefir, sauerkraut, and kimchi. Probiotics promote a healthy gut microbiome, which is crucial for digestion and overall gut health.

- Lean Proteins: Opt for lean protein sources like poultry, fish, beans, and tofu. These proteins are easier to digest and can help maintain balanced blood sugar levels.

- Limit Trigger Foods: Reduce or eliminate spicy, acidic, and fatty foods that can exacerbate acidity. Common triggers include citrus fruits, tomatoes, coffee, and fried foods.

- Hydration: Alongside Miracle Water, stay hydrated by drinking plenty of plain water throughout the day. Proper hydration ensures soft stool and facilitates smoother digestion.

5. Mindful Eating:

Practice mindful eating by savoring your meals and paying attention to hunger and fullness cues. Eating slowly and chewing thoroughly aids digestion and prevents overeating, which can contribute to both acidity and constipation.

6. Portion Control:

Overeating can strain the digestive system, leading to discomfort. Focus on portion control and avoid large meals close to bedtime to prevent acid reflux.

7. Adequate Sleep:

Quality sleep is essential for overall well-being, including digestive health. Aim for 7-9 hours of uninterrupted sleep each night to support optimal digestion.

8. Avoid Smoking and Alcohol:

Both smoking and excessive alcohol consumption can exacerbate acidity and disrupt digestion. Quit smoking and limit alcohol intake to promote better gastrointestinal health.

9. Consult a Healthcare Professional:

If your symptoms of acidity or constipation are persistent or severe, it's essential to consult a healthcare professional. They can provide personalized guidance, recommend appropriate treatments, and rule out underlying medical conditions.

10. Maintain Consistency:

Holistic approaches take time to yield noticeable results. Consistency is key. Make gradual changes to your lifestyle and dietary habits, and be patient as you await improvements in your digestive health.

Conclusion:

Chapter 6 underscores the power of a holistic approach to managing acidity and constipation. By combining the potential benefits of Miracle Water with stress management, exercise, and a balanced diet, individuals can create a comprehensive strategy for achieving optimal digestive health. Remember that each person's body is unique, so it's important to tailor these recommendations to your individual needs and preferences. By embracing these lifestyle and dietary changes, you'll be taking significant steps towards promoting a harmonious relationship between your digestive system and overall well-being.

CHAPTER 7

Case Studies and Success Stories: While you've mentioned excluding case studies, brief anecdotes or success stories could be used to illustrate the effectiveness of Miracle Water. Focus on showcasing how individuals have found relief from acidity and constipation through its use.

Case Studies and Success Stories,
Chapter 7

This chapter will explore a number of succinct examples and success stories that demonstrate Miracle Water's potential efficacy in treating constipation and acidity. These true stories provide motivational examples of how people have benefited from adding Miracle Water into their everyday routines, even though they are not comprehensive case studies.

First Anecdote: Maria's Path to Digestive Equilibrium

Maria, an office manager of 42 years, had been struggling with chronic acidity for many years. She tried a number of over-the-counter drugs, but her symptoms continued to interfere with her day-to-day activities. Maria chose to give Miracle Water a try since she found it intriguing. She began consuming a glass of Miracle Water first thing in the morning, without food. She saw a noticeable decrease in her acid reflux attacks over the course of a few weeks. Maria said, "It seems like a calming potion for my tummy. It's been years since I've felt this at ease."

Second Story: Mark Overcame Constipation

The 30-year-old fitness enthusiast Mark suffered from bloating and inconsistent bowel movements. Due to his rigorous training regimen, he frequently experienced dehydration and constipation. Mark started sipping Miracle Water following his nightly workouts as a natural treatment. He felt lighter and had better bowel regularity within weeks. "It feels like my body has found its rhythm again," remarked Mark. How something so basic has made such a difference astounds me."

Sarah's Dual Relief: Anecdote 3

The 55-year-old retiree Sarah had struggled with constipation and acidity, which caused discomfort and disturbed sleep. She chose to incorporate Miracle Water into her daily regimen since she was eager to find a comprehensive solution. After taking it twice daily, Sarah saw a progressive reduction in her symptoms of constipation and acid reflux. She said she felt less bothered by stomach problems and more energised. Sarah grinned and said, "Miracle Water has become my secret weapon for a happier gut."

Anecdote 4: John's Well-Being

John, a 37-year-old software engineer, had long had difficulty striking a balance between his occasionally excessive consumption of rich meals and his sedentary work life. His erratic feeding patterns frequently caused acidity. John was intrigued with Miracle Water and started implementing it into his regular regimen. After consuming it consistently, he noticed a considerable decrease in his acidity episodes. Furthermore, drinking Miracle Water acted as a reminder to choose better foods throughout the day.

Story 5: Emma's Path to Holistic Health

Emma was a 28-year-old yoga instructor who trusted in the efficacy of home cures. Her periodic acidity was something she tried to deal with naturally, without taking any pills. Emma began using Miracle Water as part of her daily mindfulness regimen, combining it with her yoga practice in the morning. She gradually noticed a reduction in the discomfort in her digestive tract and an improvement in her general well-being. "Miracle Water fits in well with my all-natural approach to wellness, and I appreciate the comfort it provides," said Emma.

Rendering:

These testimonials and success stories, albeit brief case studies, provide some insight into the possible advantages of Miracle Water for reducing acidity and constipation. Every person's experience is different, and their stories demonstrate the beneficial effects that little lifestyle adjustments, like consuming Miracle Water, may have on digestive health. These success stories—which demonstrate how people have used Miracle Water to enhance their everyday lives and find relief—should serve as an inspiration for you as you continue researching this natural cure.

CHAPTER 8

Frequently Asked Questions and Troubleshooting: Compile a list of common questions readers might have about Miracle Water, acidity, and constipation. Address concerns, potential challenges, and offer practical solutions to ensure a successful experience for your readers.

Naturally, readers will have questions and run into difficulties when they set out to investigate the possible advantages of Miracle Water for treating constipation and acidity. This chapter presents a thorough list of commonly asked questions (FAQs) together with helpful answers to allay worries, clear up confusion, and guarantee a successful and well-informed experience.

A1: Describe Miracle Water in detail.

A1: Alkaline and rich in minerals, Miracle Water is typically derived from natural springs or mineral water. Because of its mineral makeup and alkaline nature, it may be helpful in controlling acidity and constipation.

Q2: Can Miracle Water totally take the place of prescription drugs for constipation and acid reflux? A2: Although Miracle Water might have advantages, you should always speak with a doctor before altering your prescription schedule. They can offer you advice on how to include Miracle Water into your current treatment strategy.

Q3: What is the recommended daily intake of Miracle Water? A3: Try to consume roughly 8 glasses (or 2 liters) of water daily, including Miracle Water. In order to maintain intestinal health and stay properly hydrated, space out your intake throughout the day.

Q4: Is it okay to drink Miracle Water on an empty stomach? A4: Sure, there are advantages to doing so. It may lessen acidity symptoms by promoting a pH equilibrium and neutralizing stomach acid.

Q5: When is the optimum time to consume Miracle Water to get the greatest effects? A5: While there isn't a hard-and-fast rule, starting your day with a glass of Miracle Water in the morning will help maintain your digestive system and help you stay hydrated.

Q6: How long before I get effects from Miracle Water? A6: Everybody experiences different results. While some people may see benefits in a couple of weeks, others may require more time. Remember that consistency is essential, so keep adding Miracle Water to your regimen.

Q7: Does Miracle Water have any side effects? A7: Miracle Water is generally safe for the majority of people. Nonetheless, there may be a brief period of adjustment for certain individuals as their bodies adjust to the altered levels of hydration and mineral consumption. Seek medical advice from an expert if you encounter any strange symptoms.

Q8: Is it okay for me to drink Miracle Water while pregnant or while nursing? A8: Before making any dietary changes, including drinking Miracle Water, while pregnant or nursing, speak with your doctor.

Q9: What lifestyle modifications can augment the advantages of Miracle Water? A9: Modest lifestyle modifications, like stress reduction, consistent exercise, a balanced diet, mindful eating, and enough sleep, can complement Miracle Water's potential advantages for better digestive health.

Q10: What should I do if my symptoms don't get better? A10: If your symptoms don't get better, you might want to reconsider your diet and way of life in general. Speak with a medical expert to get specific advice and to rule out any underlying medical concerns.

Q11: Is Miracle Water safe for kids to drink? A11: Generally speaking, kids can drink Miracle Water in moderation. However, before making any dietary modifications for a child, get their pediatrician's advice.

Q12: Is it possible to create Miracle Water at home? A12: The potential health advantages of Miracle Water are enhanced by the distinctive mineral compositions found in natural springs. Although you might try adding baking soda to water to make it more alkaline, it could be difficult to make a perfect duplicate of Miracle Water.

Q13: What happens if I become more thirsty after drinking Miracle Water? A13: Getting thirstier could mean that your body is getting more hydration. When you feel thirsty, pay attention to your body and drink water. You can also add Miracle Water to this.

When using Miracle Water, may I keep taking over-the-counter antacids? A14: You can certainly keep taking antacids as needed. Seek advice from a healthcare expert, nonetheless, for help on combining the two methods.

Q15: What should I do if drinking Miracle Water causes me to have negative side effects? A15: Stop drinking Miracle Water and see a doctor if you have any negative side effects. It's critical to respond quickly to any issues raised.

Rendering.

The most frequent queries and worries regarding Miracle Water, its advantages for acidity and constipation, and its application in day-to-day living are covered in Chapter 8. Through the provision of useful answers and the removal of uncertainties, readers may confidently set out on their path, equipped with the knowledge necessary to make well-informed decisions regarding their digestive health. Keep in mind that each person's experience with Miracle Water is different, so paying attention to your body's signals and getting help from a professional when necessary are essential to having a positive encounter.

www.ingramcontent.com/pod-product-compliance
Lightning Source LLC
Chambersburg PA
CBHW050739260726
48661CB00001B/321